TYPE 2 DIABETES FOOD LIST

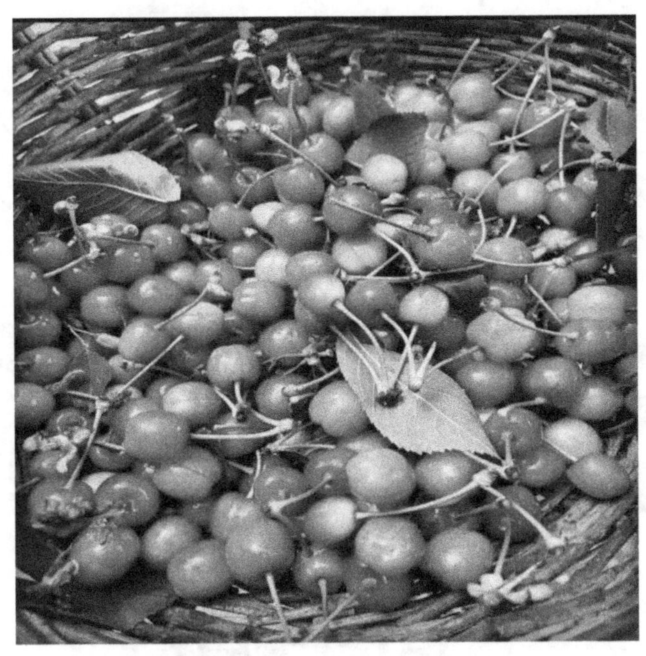

LORENE PEACHEY

DISCLAIMER

The content within this book reflects my thoughts, experiences, and beliefs. It is meant for informational and entertainment purposes. While I have taken great care to provide accurate information, I cannot guarantee the absolute correctness or applicability of the content to every individual or situation. Please consult with relevant professionals for advice specific to your needs.

TO GAIN ACCESS TO MORE BOOK BY THE AUTHOR SCAN THE QR CODE

TABLE OF CONTENTS

INTRODUCTION

In the heart of every recipe lies a story, and mine began with a quest to intertwine the tapestry of deliciousness and health. Hi there, I'm Lorene Peachey, your culinary companion on a journey to redefine what it means to eat well, especially for those dancing with the intricate steps of Type 2 Diabetes. Imagine a world where every bite is a symphony of flavor, nourishing your body while leaving your taste buds applauding in delight. That's the world I've devoted my life to creating.

For over two decades, I've navigated the labyrinth of nutritional wisdom, exploring the relationship between food and well-being. My fascination with the alchemy of ingredients began as a humble spark, fueled by a genuine desire to help individuals savor life's flavors without compromising their health.

Have you ever wondered if every meal could be a celebration of vitality? Can you envision savoring food that not only delights your palate but also nurtures your body from within? These are the questions that ignited my passion—a quest to transform the ordinary act of eating into a feast of well-being.

In my pursuit, I've encountered countless stories of triumph and resilience, individuals determined to conquer the challenges posed by Type 2 Diabetes. This is more than a mere culinary exploration; it's a journey into the very essence of life, where each recipe becomes a chapter, and every dish is a step toward vibrant health.

Picture a banquet laden with temptations – sugary treats, greasy indulgences, and a plethora of processed delights. As enticing as they may seem, these are the culprits that jeopardize the delicate dance of insulin and blood sugar levels. The consequences of such dietary recklessness are stark – the risk of cardiovascular complications, heightened blood pressure, and a body constantly grappling with inflammation.

Let me ask you this: Is it worth sacrificing your well-being for a fleeting moment of gustatory pleasure? The allure of unhealthy indulgences often masks the silent havoc they wreak on our bodies, inching us closer to a life shadowed by the complications of unmanaged diabetes.

But fear not, for my life's work has led me to uncover a trove of culinary wonders—a food list that not only tantalizes your taste buds but also champions your health. Embracing these wholesome ingredients isn't just a culinary choice; it's a lifestyle that offers a myriad of benefits.

Imagine reveling in a symphony of flavors that doesn't send your blood sugar on a roller coaster ride. Envision dishes that not only nurture your body but also bring joy to your soul. This is the promise of a well-balanced diet tailored for those with Type 2 Diabetes.

Here's the secret: the advantages of this curated food list extend far beyond blood sugar control. It's about embracing a culinary adventure that promotes overall well-being, reduces inflammation, and provides a steady stream of energy throughout the day. These recipes aren't just nourishment for your body; they're a celebration of life, a daily affirmation that health and happiness can coexist harmoniously on your plate.

In a world brimming with fad diets and conflicting nutritional advice, my mission is to simplify the journey toward a healthier you. I've meticulously crafted each recipe, drawing on the wealth of my 25-year experience as a nutritionist, to create a tapestry of flavors that aligns seamlessly with the dietary needs of those managing Type 2 Diabetes.

As you embark on this culinary odyssey with me, consider this an invitation to a world where every meal is a proclamation of self-love, a commitment to nurturing your body, mind, and spirit. Let these recipes be your compass, guiding you toward a life where wellness and culinary pleasure coalesce in a beautiful dance.

In the pages that follow, you'll discover not just recipes, but stories infused with the warmth of experience, the joy of savoring life, and the unwavering belief that every meal holds the potential to be a masterpiece of health. So, let's embark on this delicious journey together – a journey where taste knows no compromise, and well-being is the ultimate feast. Welcome to the table; the banquet of well-being awaits you.

Contact the Author

Thank you for reading my book! I would love to hear from you, whether you have feedback, questions, or just want to share your thoughts. Your feedback means a lot to me and helps me improve as a writer.

Please don't hesitate to reach out to me through

lorenepeachey@gmail.com

I look forward to connecting with my readers and appreciate your support in this literary journey. Your thoughts and comments are valuable to me.

CHAPTER 1

UNDERSTANDING TYPE 2 DIABETES

Type 2 diabetes is a chronic condition that affects how the body processes blood sugar (glucose). In individuals with this condition, the body either resists the effects of insulin—a hormone that regulates the movement of sugar into cells—or doesn't produce enough insulin to maintain normal glucose levels. As a result, blood sugar levels can become elevated, leading to various health complications.

Several factors contribute to the development of type 2 diabetes, including genetics, lifestyle choices, and environmental factors. While genetics plays a role, lifestyle modifications, particularly in diet and exercise, can significantly impact the management and prevention of type 2 diabetes.

Importance of Diet in Managing Type 2 Diabetes

Diet plays a crucial role in managing type 2 diabetes as it directly influences blood sugar levels. Making informed and healthy food choices can help regulate glucose levels, prevent complications, and improve overall well-being. Here are some key aspects of a diabetes-friendly diet:

1. **Carbohydrate Management:**

   - Focus on complex carbohydrates with a low glycemic index, such as whole grains, legumes, and vegetables.

   - Monitor portion sizes to avoid spikes in blood sugar levels.

2. **Balanced Meals:**

   - Include a combination of carbohydrates, proteins, and healthy fats in each meal.

   - This balance helps slow down the absorption of sugar and provides sustained energy.

3. **Fiber-Rich Foods:**

   - Choose foods high in fiber, such as fruits, vegetables, and whole grains.

   - Fiber helps control blood sugar levels and promotes digestive health.

4. **Limit Sugar and Processed Foods:**

   - Minimize the intake of sugary beverages, sweets, and processed foods.

   - Read food labels to identify hidden sugars and make informed choices.

5. **Healthy Fats:**

   - Opt for sources of healthy fats, such as avocados, nuts, and olive oil.

   - Limit saturated and trans fats to reduce the risk of heart disease.

6. **Regular Meal Timing:**

   - Establish a consistent eating schedule to help regulate blood sugar levels.

   - Avoid skipping meals, as this can lead to uncontrolled glucose levels.

7. **Monitoring Blood Sugar:**

- Regularly monitor blood sugar levels to understand the impact of different foods.

- Adjust dietary choices based on individual responses and recommendations from healthcare providers.

8. **Hydration:**

- Stay well-hydrated with water and limit the consumption of sugary drinks.

- Adequate hydration supports overall health and helps manage blood sugar.

CHAPTER 2

BUILDING A HEALTHY PLATE

Creating a healthy plate is a fundamental aspect of maintaining overall well-being and preventing various health conditions, including obesity and chronic diseases. The key components of building a healthy plate include portion control, balancing macronutrients, and incorporating an adequate amount of fiber.

1. **Portion Control:**

    - Be mindful of portion sizes to avoid overeating. Use smaller plates to help control portions visually.

    - Pay attention to hunger and fullness cues, and stop eating when satisfied rather than overeating.

    - Consider sharing large restaurant meals or saving part of your meal for later.

2. **Balancing Macronutrients:**

- Include a variety of macronutrients in each meal: carbohydrates, proteins, and fats.

- Carbohydrates: Choose whole grains, fruits, and vegetables for complex carbohydrates that provide sustained energy.

- Proteins: Include lean sources of protein such as poultry, fish, beans, and tofu to support muscle health.

- Fats: Opt for healthy fats like avocados, nuts, seeds, and olive oil, while limiting saturated and trans fats.

3. **Incorporating Fiber:**

- Choose whole, unprocessed foods rich in fiber to support digestion and overall health.

- Include a variety of fruits, vegetables, whole grains, legumes, and nuts in your diet.

- Aim for the recommended daily intake of fiber, which is approximately 25 grams for women and 38 grams for men.

4. **Colorful and Varied Vegetables:**

- Add a variety of colorful vegetables to your plate to ensure a diverse range of nutrients.

- Different vegetables provide different vitamins, minerals, and antioxidants that contribute to overall health.

5. **Mindful Eating:**

- Eat slowly and savor each bite to allow your body to recognize when it's satisfied.

- Minimize distractions, such as watching TV or using electronic devices, to focus on the eating experience.

6. **Hydration:**

- Drink water throughout the day to stay hydrated and support various bodily functions.

- Sometimes, thirst can be mistaken for hunger, so staying well-hydrated can aid in managing food intake.

7. **Meal Planning:**

- Plan meals in advance to make healthier choices and avoid relying on convenient, but often less nutritious, options.

- Consider batch cooking or preparing ingredients in advance to streamline healthy meal preparation.

8. **Limit Processed Foods:**

- Reduce the consumption of highly processed foods, which often contain excessive amounts of salt, sugar, and unhealthy fats.

- Choose whole, minimally processed foods for better nutritional value.

CHAPTER 3

LEAN PROTEINS

1. **Chicken Breast:**

   - Nutritional Information (per 3 ounces, cooked):

     - Calories: 165

     - Protein: 31g

     - Fat: 3.6g

     - Saturated Fat: 1g

     - Carbohydrates: 0g

     - Fiber: 0g

2. **Salmon:**

   - Nutritional Information (per 3 ounces, cooked):

     - Calories: 177

     - Protein: 23g

     - Fat: 9g

     - Saturated Fat: 1.3g

     - Omega-3 Fatty Acids: 1,023mg

     - Carbohydrates: 0g

3. **Tofu:**

- Nutritional Information (per 3 ounces, firm, cooked):

    - Calories: 144

    - Protein: 16g

    - Fat: 8g

    - Carbohydrates: 3g

    - Fiber: 1g

4. **Turkey Breast:**

- Nutritional Information (per 3 ounces, cooked):

    - Calories: 135

    - Protein: 30g

    - Fat: 1g

    - Saturated Fat: 0.3g

    - Carbohydrates: 0g

    - Fiber: 0g

5. **Greek Yogurt (Non-fat):**

- Nutritional Information (per 6 ounces):

    - Calories: 100

    - Protein: 15g

    - Fat: 0g

    - Carbohydrates: 6g

    - Sugar: 6g

6. **Lean Ground Beef (90% lean):**

- Nutritional Information (per 3 ounces, cooked):

    - Calories: 184

    - Protein: 21g

    - Fat: 11g

    - Saturated Fat: 4.5g

    - Carbohydrates: 0g

    - Fiber: 0g

7. **Eggs:**

- Nutritional Information (per large egg):

    - Calories: 70

    - Protein: 6g

    - Fat: 5g

    - Saturated Fat: 1.6g

    - Carbohydrates: 1g

    - Fiber: 0g

8. **Cottage Cheese (Low-fat):**

- Nutritional Information (per 1/2 cup):

    - Calories: 90

    - Protein: 14g

    - Fat: 1.5g

    - Saturated Fat: 1g

    - Carbohydrates: 4g

    - Sugar: 2g

9. **Shrimp:**

- Nutritional Information (per 3 ounces, cooked):

    - Calories: 84

    - Protein: 18g

    - Fat: 1.1g

    - Carbohydrates: 0g

    - Fiber: 0g

10. **Lean Pork Tenderloin:**

- Nutritional Information (per 3 ounces, cooked):

    - Calories: 143

    - Protein: 24g

    - Fat: 4g

    - Saturated Fat: 1.2g

    - Carbohydrates: 0g

    - Fiber: 0g

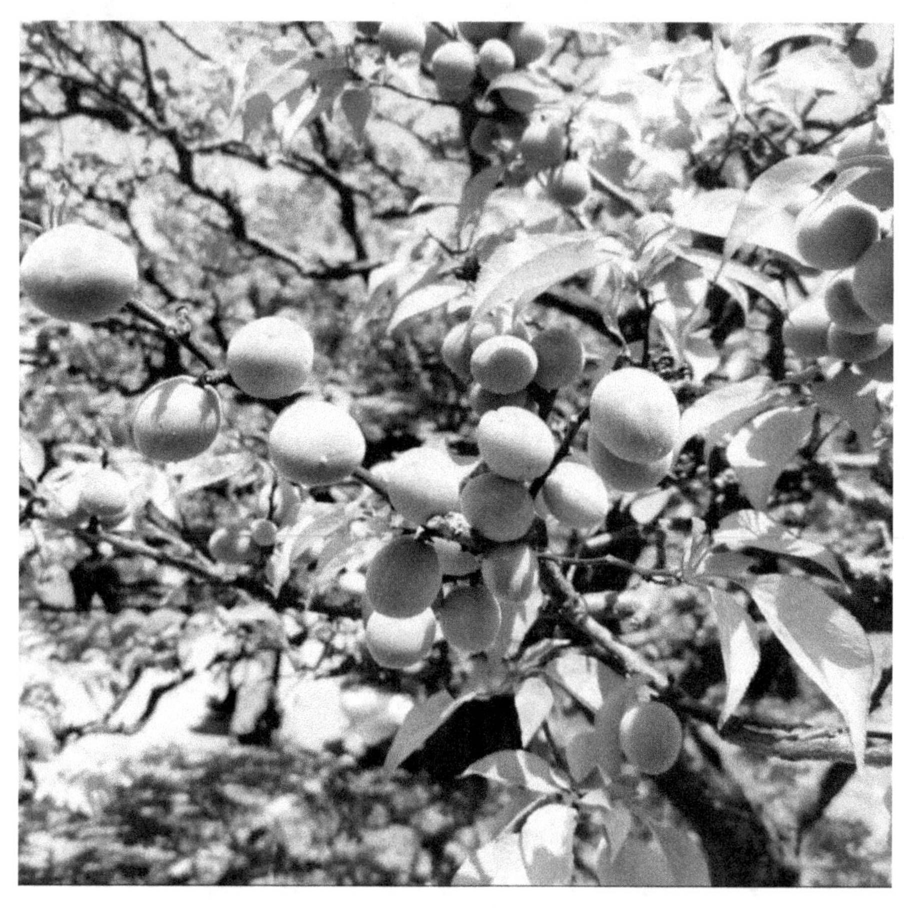

CHAPTER 4

WHOLE GRAINS

1. **Quinoa:**

    - Nutritional Information (per 1 cup, cooked):

        - Calories: 222

        - Protein: 8g

        - Fat: 4g

        - Carbohydrates: 39g

        - Fiber: 5g

2. **Brown Rice:**

    - Nutritional Information (per 1 cup, cooked):

        - Calories: 215

        - Protein: 5g

        - Fat: 1.6g

        - Carbohydrates: 45g

        - Fiber: 3.5g

3. **Oats (Old-Fashioned):**

- Nutritional Information (per 1 cup, cooked):

    - Calories: 154

    - Protein: 5g

    - Fat: 3g

    - Carbohydrates: 27g

    - Fiber: 4g

4. **Bulgur:**

- Nutritional Information (per 1 cup, cooked):

    - Calories: 151

    - Protein: 5g

    - Fat: 0.4g

    - Carbohydrates: 34g

    - Fiber: 8g

5. **Barley:**

- Nutritional Information (per 1 cup, cooked):

    - Calories: 193

    - Protein: 3.5g

    - Fat: 0.7g

    - Carbohydrates: 44g

    - Fiber: 6g

6. **Whole Wheat Pasta:**

- Nutritional Information (per 1 cup, cooked):

    - Calories: 174

    - Protein: 7.5g

    - Fat: 1.3g

    - Carbohydrates: 37g

    - Fiber: 6g

7. **Farro:**

- Nutritional Information (per 1 cup, cooked):

  - Calories: 220

  - Protein: 8g

  - Fat: 1.5g

  - Carbohydrates: 47g

  - Fiber: 7g

8. **Millet:**

- Nutritional Information (per 1 cup, cooked):

  - Calories: 207

  - Protein: 6g

  - Fat: 2g

  - Carbohydrates: 41g

  - Fiber: 2.3g

9. **Whole Wheat Bread:**

- Nutritional Information (per 1 slice):

    - Calories: 69

    - Protein: 3g

    - Fat: 1g

    - Carbohydrates: 12g

    - Fiber: 2g

10. **Wild Rice:**

- Nutritional Information (per 1 cup, cooked):

    - Calories: 166

    - Protein: 6.5g

    - Fat: 0.6g

    - Carbohydrates: 35g

    - Fiber: 3g

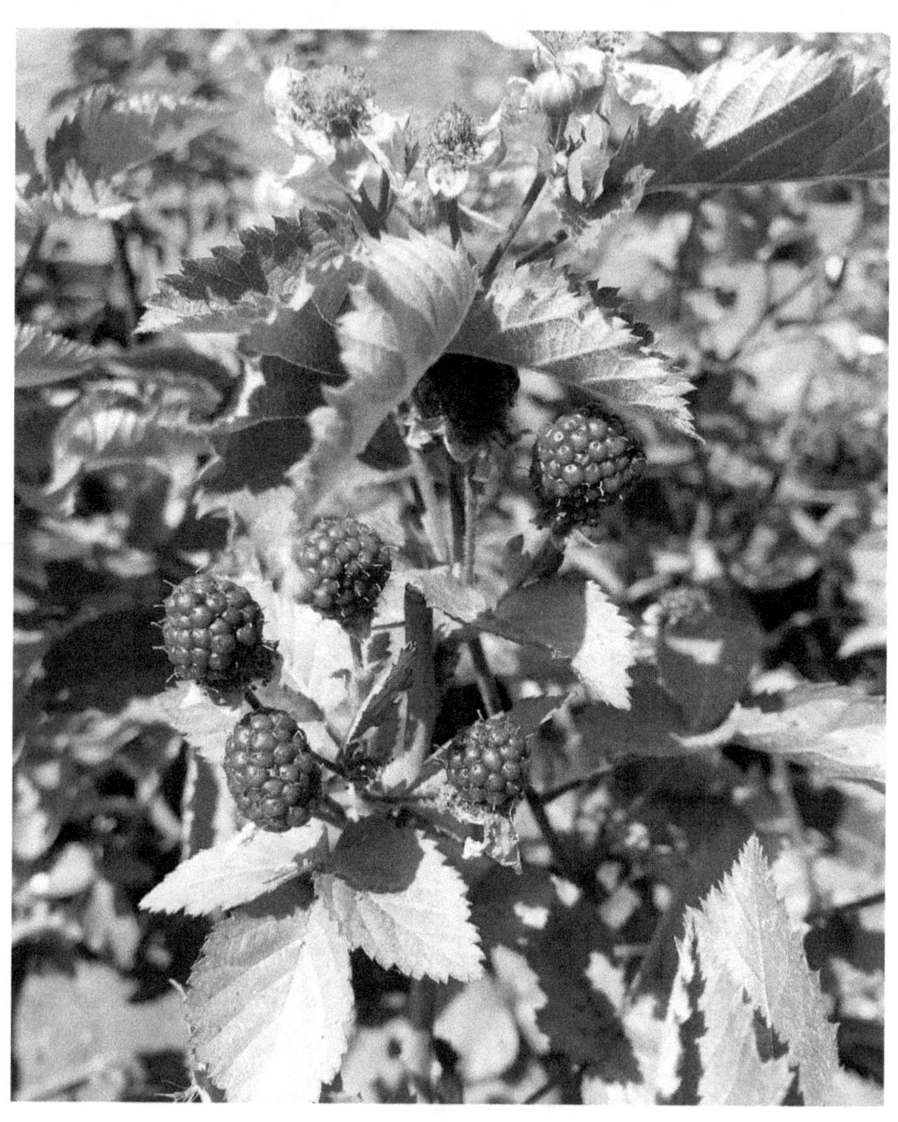

CHAPTER 5
FRUITS

1. **Berries (Blueberries):**

   - Nutritional Information (per 1 cup, fresh):

     - Calories: 84

     - Carbohydrates: 21g

     - Fiber: 4g

     - Sugars: 15g

     - Vitamin C: 14mg

2. **Apples:**

   - Nutritional Information (per medium apple):

     - Calories: 95

     - Carbohydrates: 25g

     - Fiber: 4g

     - Sugars: 19g

     - Vitamin C: 14% of daily recommended intake

3. **Cherries:**

- Nutritional Information (per 1 cup, fresh):

    - Calories: 87

    - Carbohydrates: 22g

    - Fiber: 3g

    - Sugars: 18g

    - Vitamin C: 10mg

4. **Grapes:**

- Nutritional Information (per 1 cup, seedless):

    - Calories: 104

    - Carbohydrates: 27g

    - Fiber: 1g

    - Sugars: 23g

    - Vitamin C: 4mg

5. **Pears:**

- Nutritional Information (per medium pear):

    - Calories: 101

    - Carbohydrates: 27g

    - Fiber: 6g

    - Sugars: 17g

    - Vitamin C: 7mg

6. **Strawberries:**

- Nutritional Information (per 1 cup, fresh):

    - Calories: 50

    - Carbohydrates: 11g

    - Fiber: 3g

    - Sugars: 7g

    - Vitamin C: 89mg

7. **Oranges:**

- Nutritional Information (per medium orange):

    - Calories: 62

    - Carbohydrates: 15g

    - Fiber: 3g

    - Sugars: 12g

    - Vitamin C: 70mg

8. **Kiwi:**

- Nutritional Information (per medium kiwi):

    - Calories: 61

    - Carbohydrates: 15g

    - Fiber: 3g

    - Sugars: 9g

    - Vitamin C: 71mg

9. **Plums:**

- Nutritional Information (per 2 medium plums):

    - Calories: 60

    - Carbohydrates: 16g

    - Fiber: 2g

    - Sugars: 12g

    - Vitamin C: 16mg

10. **Peaches:**

- Nutritional Information (per medium peach):

    - Calories: 58

    - Carbohydrates: 14g

    - Fiber: 2g

    - Sugars: 13g

    - Vitamin C: 7mg

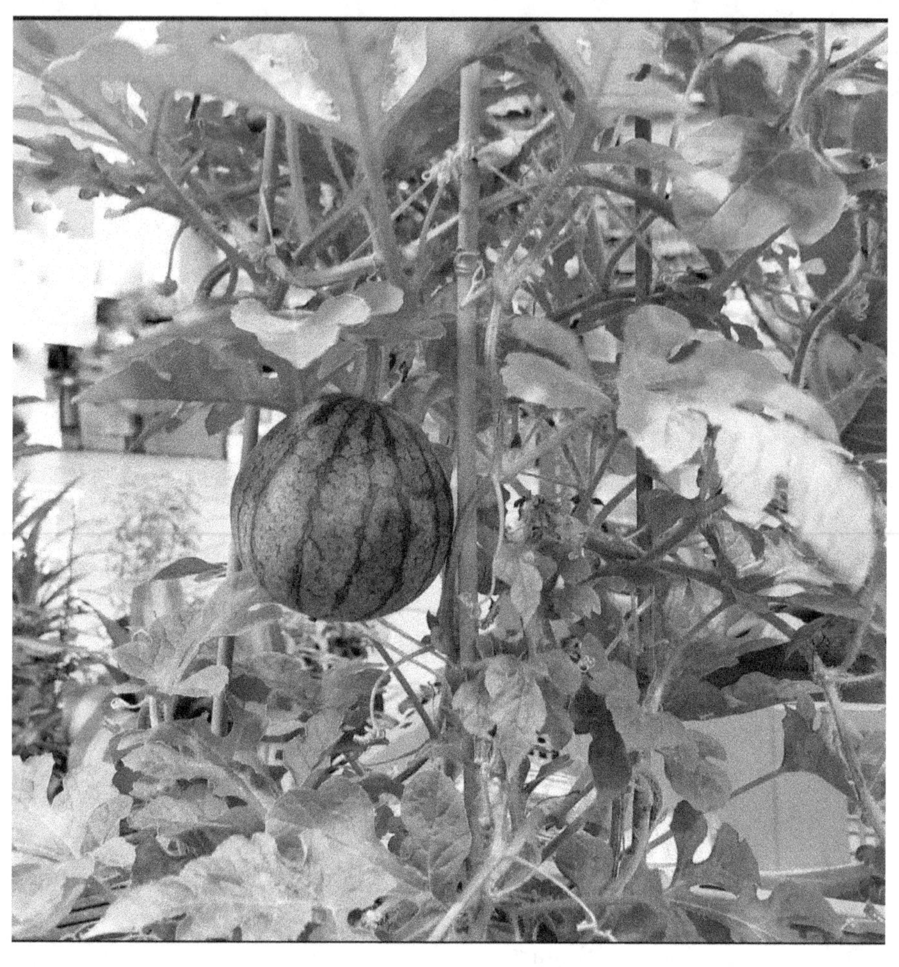

CHAPTER 6

VEGETABLES

1. **Broccoli:**

    - Nutritional Information (per 1 cup, cooked):

        - Calories: 55

        - Carbohydrates: 11g

        - Fiber: 5g

        - Protein: 3.7g

        - Vitamin C: 81mg

2. **Spinach:**

    - Nutritional Information (per 1 cup, cooked):

        - Calories: 41

        - Carbohydrates: 6.7g

        - Fiber: 4.7g

        - Protein: 5.4g

        - Vitamin A: 9432 IU

3. **Cauliflower:**

- Nutritional Information (per 1 cup, raw):

    - Calories: 27

    - Carbohydrates: 5.3g

    - Fiber: 2.5g

    - Protein: 2g

    - Vitamin C: 51mg

4. **Carrots:**

- Nutritional Information (per 1 cup, raw):

    - Calories: 52

    - Carbohydrates: 12g

    - Fiber: 3.6g

    - Protein: 1.2g

    - Vitamin A: 509% of daily recommended intake

5. **Bell Peppers (Red):**

- Nutritional Information (per 1 cup, raw):

    - Calories: 46

    - Carbohydrates: 9g

    - Fiber: 3g

    - Protein: 1.5g

    - Vitamin C: 212mg

6. **Zucchini:**

- Nutritional Information (per 1 cup, raw):

    - Calories: 20

    - Carbohydrates: 4g

    - Fiber: 1.5g

    - Protein: 1.4g

    - Vitamin C: 21mg

7. **Brussels Sprouts:**

- Nutritional Information (per 1 cup, cooked):

    - Calories: 56

    - Carbohydrates: 12g

    - Fiber: 4g

    - Protein: 4g

    - Vitamin C: 75mg

8. **Cabbage:**

- Nutritional Information (per 1 cup, shredded):

    - Calories: 22

    - Carbohydrates: 5g

    - Fiber: 2g

    - Protein: 1g

    - Vitamin C: 28mg

9. **Asparagus:**

- Nutritional Information (per 1 cup, cooked):

    - Calories: 32

    - Carbohydrates: 6g

    - Fiber: 2.8g

    - Protein: 3g

    - Vitamin C: 8mg

10. **Kale:**

- Nutritional Information (per 1 cup, raw):

    - Calories: 33

    - Carbohydrates: 6g

    - Fiber: 1.3g

    - Protein: 2.2g

    - Vitamin A: 6699 IU

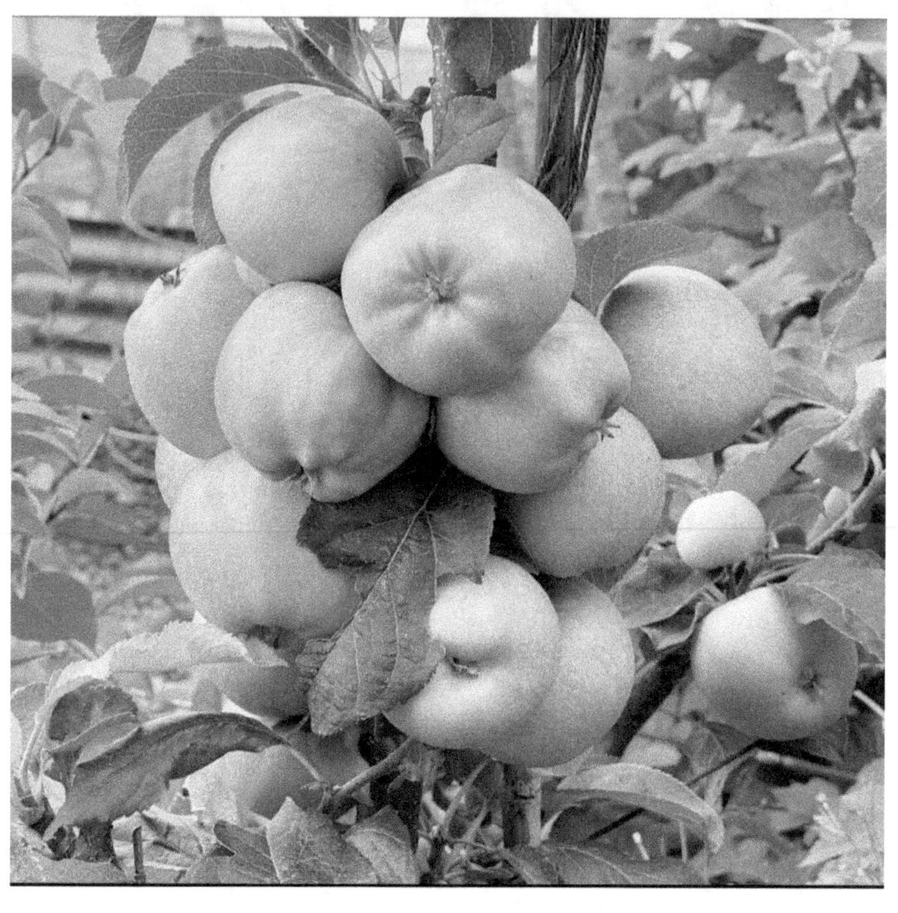

CHAPTER 7

FOODS TO LIMIT OR AVOID

1. **Sugar-Sweetened Beverages:**

   - Nutritional Information (per 12-ounce can of cola):

     - Calories: 140

     - Sugars: 39g

2. **Candy and Sweets:**

   - Nutritional Information (per standard chocolate bar):

     - Calories: Varies (typically 200-300 calories)

     - Sugars: Varies (typically 20-30g)

3. **Processed Snack Foods (Chips, Crackers):**

   - Nutritional Information (per 1 ounce of potato chips):

     - Calories: 152

     - Carbohydrates: 15g

     - Saturated Fat: 1.4g

     - Sodium: 152mg

4. **White Bread and Refined Grains:**

- Nutritional Information (per 2 slices of white bread):

    - Calories: 140

    - Carbohydrates: 28g

    - Fiber: 1g

5. **French Fries and Fried Foods:**

- Nutritional Information (per medium serving of fast-food fries):

    - Calories: 365

    - Carbohydrates: 63g

    - Total Fat: 14g

    - Sodium: 246mg

6. **Regular Pasta:**

- Nutritional Information (per 1 cup, cooked):

    - Calories: 200

    - Carbohydrates: 40g

    - Fiber: 2g

7. **Sweetened Breakfast Cereals:**

- Nutritional Information (per 1 cup of a sweetened cereal):

    - Calories: Varies (typically 100-200 calories)

    - Sugars: Varies (typically 10-20g)

8. **Fruit Juices and Sweetened Drinks:**

- Nutritional Information (per 8 ounces of orange juice):

    - Calories: 110

    - Sugars: 21g

9. **High-Fat Processed Meats (Sausages, Bacon):**

- Nutritional Information (per 3 slices of bacon):

    - Calories: 135

    - Total Fat: 12g

    - Saturated Fat: 4g

10. **Full-Fat Dairy Products:**

- Nutritional Information (per 1 cup of whole milk):

    - Calories: 150

    - Total Fat: 8g

    - Saturated Fat: 5g

CHAPTER 8

RECIPES FOR TYPE 2 DIABETES

Breakfast Ideas

Veggie Omelette with Whole Grain Toast

Cooking Time: 10 minutes

Servings: 1

Ingredients:

- 2 large eggs

- 1/4 cup bell peppers, diced

- 1/4 cup tomatoes, diced

- 1/4 cup spinach, chopped

- Salt and pepper to taste

- 2 slices of whole grain bread

Instructions:

1. Whisk eggs in a bowl and season with salt and pepper.

2. Mix in bell peppers, tomatoes, and spinach.

3. Pour mixture into a heated, non-stick skillet.

4. Cook until the edges set, then flip and cook the other side.

5. Toast whole grain bread slices.

6. Serve the omelette over the toast.

Nutritional Information: (Per Serving) Calories: 280 | Protein: 18g | Carbohydrates: 22g | Fiber: 5g | Fat: 14g

Greek Yogurt Parfait with Berries and Almonds

Cooking Time: 5 minutes

Servings: 1

Ingredients:

- 1 cup Greek yogurt (non-fat)

- 1/2 cup mixed berries (blueberries, strawberries)

- 2 tablespoons almonds, chopped

- 1 teaspoon honey (optional)

Instructions:

1. In a glass, layer Greek yogurt, mixed berries, and chopped almonds.

2. Repeat layers until the glass is filled.

3. Drizzle with honey if desired.

Nutritional Information: (Per Serving) Calories: 280 | Protein: 20g | Carbohydrates: 25g | Fiber: 4g | Fat: 12g

Avocado and Tomato Toast

Cooking Time: 5 minutes

Servings: 1

Ingredients:

- 1 ripe avocado

- 1 medium tomato, sliced

- 2 slices whole grain bread

- Salt and pepper to taste

- Optional: red pepper flakes, for added spice

Instructions:

1. Toast whole grain bread slices.

2. Mash the avocado and spread it evenly on the toasted bread.

3. Top with tomato slices and season with salt, pepper, and red pepper flakes if desired.

Nutritional Information: (Per Serving) Calories: 320 | Protein: 8g | Carbohydrates: 35g | Fiber: 12g | Fat: 18g

Overnight Oats with Chia Seeds and Berries

Prep Time: 5 minutes (plus overnight soaking)

Servings: 1

Ingredients:

- 1/2 cup rolled oats

- 1/2 cup unsweetened almond milk

- 1 tablespoon chia seeds

- 1/2 cup mixed berries (strawberries, blueberries)

- 1 tablespoon almond butter

- 1 teaspoon honey (optional)

Instructions:

1. In a jar, combine rolled oats, almond milk, and chia seeds.

2. Stir well, cover, and refrigerate overnight.

3. In the morning, top with mixed berries, almond butter, and a drizzle of honey if desired.

Nutritional Information: (Per Serving) Calories: 350 | Protein: 10g | Carbohydrates: 48g | Fiber: 12g | Fat: 15g

Vegetable and Cheese Breakfast Wrap

Cooking Time: 15 minutes

Servings: 1

Ingredients:

- 1 whole-grain tortilla

- 2 large eggs, scrambled

- 1/4 cup bell peppers, diced

- 1/4 cup onions, diced

- 1/4 cup cherry tomatoes, halved

- 1/4 cup shredded low-fat cheese

- Salt and pepper to taste

- Fresh herbs (e.g., parsley) for garnish

Instructions:

1. In a non-stick pan, sauté bell peppers and onions until softened.

2. Add scrambled eggs, cherry tomatoes, salt, and pepper. Cook until eggs are set.

3. Warm the tortilla and place the egg mixture on it.

4. Sprinkle shredded cheese on top and fold into a wrap.

5. Garnish with fresh herbs and serve.

Nutritional Information: (Per Serving) Calories: 380 | Protein: 25g | Carbohydrates: 30g | Fiber: 6g | Fat: 18g

Lunch and Dinner Recipes

Grilled Chicken Salad with Quinoa

Cooking Time: 30 minutes

Servings: 2

Ingredients:

- 2 boneless, skinless chicken breasts

- 1 cup quinoa, cooked

- 4 cups mixed salad greens

- 1 cup cherry tomatoes, halved

- 1/2 cucumber, sliced

- 1/4 cup feta cheese, crumbled

- 2 tablespoons olive oil

- 1 tablespoon balsamic vinegar

- Salt and pepper to taste

Instructions:

1. Season chicken breasts with salt and pepper, then grill until fully cooked.

2. In a bowl, combine cooked quinoa, salad greens, cherry tomatoes, cucumber, and feta cheese.

3. Slice grilled chicken and place on top of the salad.

4. In a small bowl, whisk together olive oil and balsamic vinegar, then drizzle over the salad.

Nutritional Information: (Per Serving) Calories: 480 | Protein: 35g | Carbohydrates: 40g | Fiber: 6g | Fat: 20g

Baked Salmon with Roasted Vegetables

Cooking Time: 25 minutes

Servings: 2

Ingredients:

- 2 salmon fillets

- 1 cup broccoli florets

- 1 cup carrots, sliced

- 1 cup cherry tomatoes

- 2 tablespoons olive oil

- 1 teaspoon garlic powder

- 1 teaspoon dried thyme

- Salt and pepper to taste

- Lemon wedges for serving

Instructions:

1. Preheat oven to 400°F (200°C).

2. Place salmon fillets on a baking sheet lined with parchment paper.

3. In a bowl, toss broccoli, carrots, and cherry tomatoes with olive oil, garlic powder, thyme, salt, and pepper.

4. Spread the vegetable mixture around the salmon on the baking sheet.

5. Bake for 20-25 minutes or until salmon is cooked through and vegetables are tender.

6. Serve with lemon wedges.

Nutritional Information: (Per Serving) Calories: 420 | Protein: 35g | Carbohydrates: 15g | Fiber: 5g | Fat: 25g

Turkey and Vegetable Stir-Fry with Brown Rice

Cooking Time: 20 minutes

Servings: 3

Ingredients:

- 1 pound lean ground turkey

- 2 cups broccoli florets

- 1 bell pepper, sliced

- 1 cup snap peas

- 2 tablespoons low-sodium soy sauce

- 1 tablespoon sesame oil

- 1 tablespoon ginger, minced

- 2 cloves garlic, minced

- 2 cups cooked brown rice

Instructions:

1. In a large skillet, brown ground turkey over medium heat.

2. Add broccoli, bell pepper, and snap peas to the skillet and stir-fry for 5-7 minutes.

3. In a small bowl, mix soy sauce, sesame oil, ginger, and garlic. Pour over the turkey and vegetables.

4. Continue cooking until vegetables are tender.

5. Serve the stir-fry over cooked brown rice.

Nutritional Information: (Per Serving) Calories: 380 | Protein: 30g | Carbohydrates: 40g | Fiber: 6g | Fat: 12g

Quinoa and Black Bean Stuffed Peppers

Cooking Time: 40 minutes

Servings: 4

Ingredients:

- 4 large bell peppers, halved and seeds removed

- 1 cup quinoa, cooked

- 1 can (15 oz) black beans, drained and rinsed

- 1 cup corn kernels (fresh or frozen)

- 1 cup cherry tomatoes, diced

- 1 teaspoon cumin

- 1 teaspoon chili powder

- 1/2 teaspoon garlic powder

- Salt and pepper to taste

- 1 cup shredded low-fat cheese (optional)

Instructions:

1. Preheat oven to 375°F (190°C).

2. In a large bowl, mix quinoa, black beans, corn, cherry tomatoes, cumin, chili powder, garlic powder, salt, and pepper.

3. Spoon the mixture into halved bell peppers and place in a baking dish.

4. If desired, sprinkle shredded cheese on top.

5. Cover with foil and bake for 30 minutes. Remove foil and bake for an additional 10 minutes until peppers are tender.

Nutritional Information: (Per Serving) Calories: 320 | Protein: 15g | Carbohydrates: 55g | Fiber: 11g | Fat: 4g

Lentil and Vegetable Soup

Cooking Time: 45 minutes

Servings: 6

Ingredients:

- 1 cup dried green or brown lentils, rinsed

- 1 onion, diced

- 2 carrots, diced

- 2 celery stalks, diced

- 3 cloves garlic, minced

- 1 can (14 oz) diced tomatoes

- 6 cups vegetable broth (low-sodium)

- 1 teaspoon cumin

- 1 teaspoon paprika

- 1/2 teaspoon turmeric

- Salt and pepper to taste

- 2 cups kale, chopped

Instructions:

1. In a large pot, sauté onion, carrots, and celery until softened.

2. Add garlic and sauté for an additional 1-2 minutes.

3. Stir in lentils, diced tomatoes, vegetable broth, cumin, paprika, turmeric, salt, and pepper.

4. Bring to a boil, then reduce heat and simmer for 30-35 minutes or until lentils are tender.

5. Add chopped kale and cook for an additional 5 minutes.

Nutritional Information: (Per Serving) Calories: 220 | Protein: 13g | Carbohydrates: 40g | Fiber: 10g | Fat: 1g

Snack Options

Greek Yogurt and Berry Parfait

Preparation Time: 5 minutes

Servings: 1

Ingredients:

- 1 cup Greek yogurt (non-fat)
- 1/2 cup mixed berries (blueberries, strawberries)
- 2 tablespoons almonds, chopped
- 1 teaspoon honey (optional)

Instructions:

1. In a tall glass or a bowl, start by layering 1/4 cup of Greek yogurt.

2. Add a layer of 2 tablespoons of mixed berries.

3. Sprinkle 1 tablespoon of chopped almonds over the berries.

4. Repeat the layering process until the glass is filled.

5. Drizzle with honey if desired.

6. Use a long spoon to enjoy each layer.

Nutritional Information: (Per Serving) Calories: 280 | Protein: 20g | Carbohydrates: 25g | Fiber: 4g | Fat: 12g

Veggie Sticks with Hummus

Preparation Time: 10 minutes

Servings: 2

Ingredients:

- 1 cup baby carrots

- 1 cup cucumber, sliced

- 1 cup cherry tomatoes

- 1/2 cup hummus

Instructions:

1. Wash and prepare the vegetables by cutting baby carrots, cucumber, and cherry tomatoes.

2. Arrange the veggie sticks on a plate.

3. Place the hummus in a bowl for dipping.

4. Dip the veggie sticks into the hummus and enjoy.

Nutritional Information: (Per Serving) Calories: 120 | Protein: 4g | Carbohydrates: 15g | Fiber: 6g | Fat: 6g

Hard-Boiled Egg and Whole Grain Crackers

Preparation Time: 15 minutes

Servings: 2

Ingredients:

- 2 hard-boiled eggs, sliced

- 1 cup whole grain crackers

- Salt and pepper to taste

Instructions:

1. Boil eggs until fully cooked, peel, and slice them.

2. Arrange the hard-boiled egg slices on a plate.

3. Serve with a cup of whole grain crackers.

4. Season with salt and pepper according to taste.

Nutritional Information: (Per Serving) Calories: 220 | Protein: 12g | Carbohydrates: 25g | Fiber: 4g | Fat: 8g

Apple Slices with Almond Butter

Preparation Time: 5 minutes

Servings: 1

Ingredients:

- 1 medium apple, sliced

- 2 tablespoons almond butter

Instructions:

1. Wash and slice the apple into wedges.

2. Place the apple slices on a plate.

3. In a small bowl, serve 2 tablespoons of almond butter for dipping.

4. Dip the apple slices into the almond butter and enjoy.

Nutritional Information: (Per Serving) Calories: 230 | Protein: 3g | Carbohydrates: 30g | Fiber: 5g | Fat: 13g

Cottage Cheese and Pineapple Bowl

Preparation Time: 5 minutes

Servings: 1

Ingredients:

- 1 cup low-fat cottage cheese

- 1/2 cup pineapple chunks (fresh or canned, in natural juice)

Instructions:

1. In a bowl, scoop 1 cup of low-fat cottage cheese.

2. Add 1/2 cup of pineapple chunks on top.

3. Mix gently and enjoy the combination of cottage cheese and pineapple.

Nutritional Information: (Per Serving) Calories: 220 | Protein: 28g | Carbohydrates: 20g | Fiber: 2g | Fat: 3.5g

CONCLUSION

As we approach the final chapter of this culinary odyssey, I invite you to reflect on the flavors we've explored, the stories we've uncovered, and the transformative power each recipe holds. The kitchen, once a place of mere sustenance, has become a canvas for crafting a life infused with health, joy, and a celebration of the senses.

Together, we've ventured into the realm of Type 2 Diabetes management, weaving a tapestry of recipes designed not only to regulate blood sugar levels but to elevate your dining experience. This isn't just a collection of dishes; it's a testament to the potential that lies within every ingredient, every mindful bite.

As you embark on the journey ahead, consider this more than a culinary exploration—it's an ongoing narrative of well-being. The recipes within these pages are not confined to the kitchen; they are companions on your journey to sustained health. May each meal be a proclamation that you are the steward of your own vitality, and every ingredient is a brushstroke in the masterpiece of your well-being.

Remember, progress is a journey, not a destination. The recipes you've discovered here are mere stepping stones toward a life where wellness isn't a fleeting concept but a daily celebration. Small changes compound into significant transformations, and with each nutritious choice, you're investing in a healthier, more vibrant you.

As our culinary adventure concludes, I extend an earnest invitation for your feedback. Your thoughts, experiences, and suggestions are invaluable. Did a particular recipe become a staple in your kitchen? How did the flavors resonate with you? Your insights can shape the future, guiding the creation of more tailored recipes and fostering a community united by a commitment to well-being.

Feel free to share your journey on my email, and let our community thrive on shared successes, challenges, and the joy found in every bite. Your feedback isn't just welcomed; it's an integral part of the ongoing conversation about health, happiness, and the harmonious marriage of deliciousness and nourishment.

In closing, I express my deepest gratitude for allowing me to be a part of your culinary voyage. Crafting these recipes has been a labor of love and knowing that they have found a place in your homes brings immeasurable joy. As you savor the flavors of well-being, may your journey continue to be filled with vitality, satisfaction, and the delightful dance of taste.

So, until our next culinary rendezvous, I bid you farewell with a heart full of gratitude. Bon appétit, dear friend, and may your path be sprinkled with the spices of health, happiness, and the pure joy of savoring life.

BONUS CHAPTER

EXERCISE AND NUTRITION TIPS

Regular physical activity plays a crucial role in managing blood sugar levels for individuals with diabetes. Here's how:

1. **Improved Insulin Sensitivity:** Exercise helps the body use insulin more effectively, allowing cells to take in and use glucose for energy.

2. **Weight Management:** Physical activity contributes to weight loss or maintenance, reducing the risk of insulin resistance associated with obesity.

3. **Blood Sugar Regulation:** Exercise helps lower blood sugar levels by increasing glucose uptake by muscles during and after activity.

4. **Enhanced Cardiovascular Health:** Regular exercise improves heart health, reducing the risk of cardiovascular complications often associated with diabetes.

5. **Stress Reduction:** Physical activity can lower stress levels, which can indirectly impact blood sugar levels as stress hormones can affect insulin resistance.

Pre- and Post-Exercise Nutrition:

Pre-Exercise: Consuming a balanced meal or snack before exercise is essential to provide energy and stabilize blood sugar levels. Include complex carbohydrates, lean proteins, and healthy fats.

Example Pre-Exercise Snack:

- Whole grain toast with peanut butter

- Greek yogurt with berries

- Banana with a handful of nuts

Post-Exercise: After exercise, focus on replenishing glycogen stores and promoting muscle recovery. A combination of carbohydrates and proteins is beneficial.

Example Post-Exercise Meal:

- Grilled chicken breast with quinoa and roasted vegetables

- Salmon with sweet potato and steamed broccoli

- Whole grain pasta with lean turkey meat sauce

Diabetes Exercises:

1. **Aerobic Exercise (Cardio):**

   - Activities: Walking, jogging, cycling, swimming.

   - Duration: Aim for at least 150 minutes per week of moderate-intensity aerobic exercise.

2. **Strength Training:**

   - Activities: Weightlifting, resistance band exercises.

   - Frequency: Include strength training 2-3 times per week.

3. **Flexibility Exercises:**

   - Activities: Yoga, stretching.

   - Frequency: Engage in flexibility exercises regularly to improve range of motion.

4. **Balance Training:**

   - Activities: Tai Chi, balance exercises.

   - Frequency: Include balance training 2-3 times per week.

5. **Interval Training:**

- Activities: Alternating between high-intensity and low-intensity exercise.

- Duration: Short bursts of intense activity followed by rest.

Important Tips:

- Consult with a healthcare professional before starting a new exercise program.

- Monitor blood sugar levels before and after exercise, especially in the beginning.

- Stay hydrated and carry a source of fast-acting carbohydrates during exercise in case of low blood sugar (hypoglycemia).

Remember: Individual exercise needs may vary, and it's crucial to tailor activities to personal preferences, fitness levels, and any existing health conditions. Regular communication with healthcare providers and registered dietitians ensures a comprehensive approach to diabetes management.

BONUS EMAIL CONSULTATION

Embark on a transformative wellness journey with a bonus free email consultation led by a seasoned nutritionist boasting 25 years of expertise. This exclusive opportunity invites you to delve into a personalized chapter of health, where I will share invaluable insights and tailored advice to elevate your overall well-being. Whether you seek weight management, nutritional guidance, or specific health improvements, my wealth of experience ensures a comprehensive approach to meet your unique needs.

During this consultation, we will explore your current lifestyle, dietary preferences, and wellness aspirations. By collaborating through email, I aim to provide you with a roadmap for sustainable health and vitality. Seize this chance to ask questions, address concerns, and gain a deeper understanding of how nutrition can positively impact your life. To claim your bonus chapter consultation, simply send me an email with a brief overview of your health goals, and let's kickstart your journey to a healthier, more vibrant you.

lorenepeachey@gmail.com